Nose to Toes

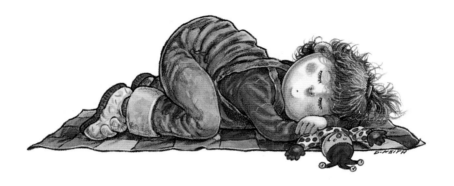

By JoAnne Nelson
Illustrated by Doug Keith

Published by
The Wright Group
19201 120th Avenue NE
Bothell, WA 98011-9512

©1995 by Comprehensive Health Education Foundation (C.H.E.F.®)
22323 Pacific Highway South
Seattle, WA 98198

Printed in Canada.

99 98 97 96 95   5 4 3 2 1

Library of Congress Cataloging-in-Publication Data
Nelson, JoAnne
        Nose to Toes / by JoAnne Nelson; illustrated by Doug Keith
        p. cm.
        Summary: Rhyming text introduces the skin and the muscular and skeletal systems
        of the human body.
        1. Musculoskeletal system—Juvenile literature. 2. Skin—Juvenile literature
        [1. Skin. 2. Muscular system. 3. Skeleton.]
        I. Keith, Doug. ill. II Title.
        OM100.N45 1992 611'.7—dc 20

ISBN: 0-7802-3245-3   CIP 91-34706
ISBN: 0-7802-3106-6 (6-pack)

This is the me that you can see.
But there's so much more

inside of me!

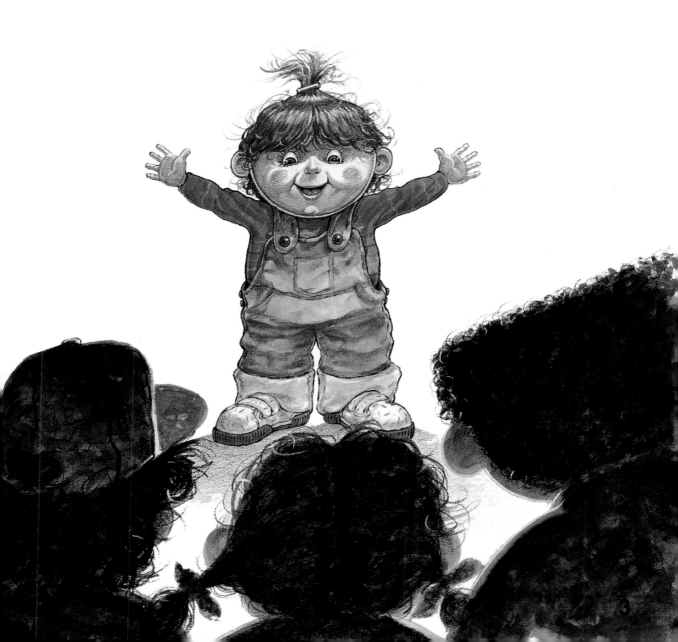

Skin covers me
from my head to my toes,
from the tip of my fingers
to the tip of my nose.

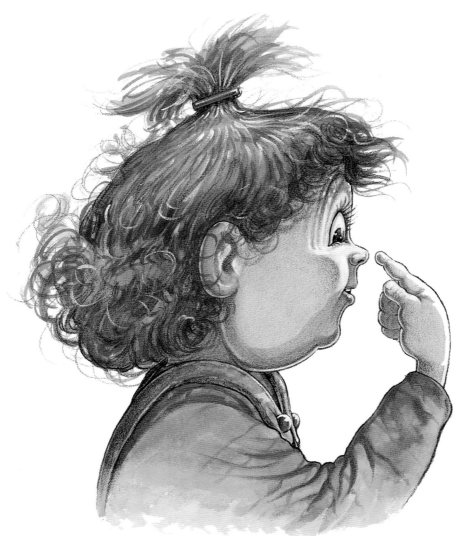

My skin keeps me warm.
My skin keeps me cool.
But when it's really hot,
I cool off in the pool.

When I get hot, tiny pores in my skin open, and sweat comes out.
I feel cooler as the air dries my skin.
When it's cold, my pores close tight.

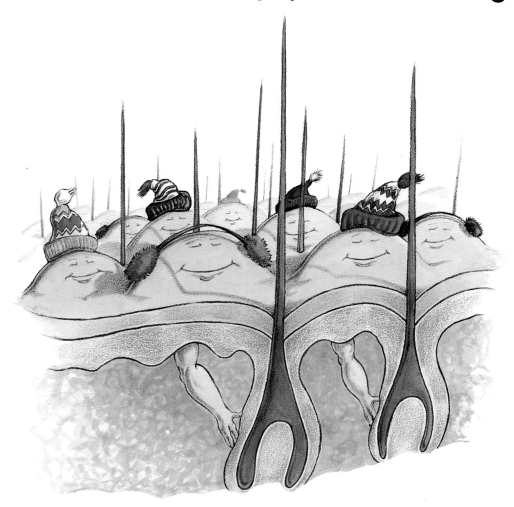

Tiny muscles make the hair
on my skin stand up straight
and make "goose bumps"
under my skin.

My skin is tough—but sometimes
it's not tough enough!
When I get cut or get a bump,
I sometimes bleed or get a lump.
Then my body heals itself!

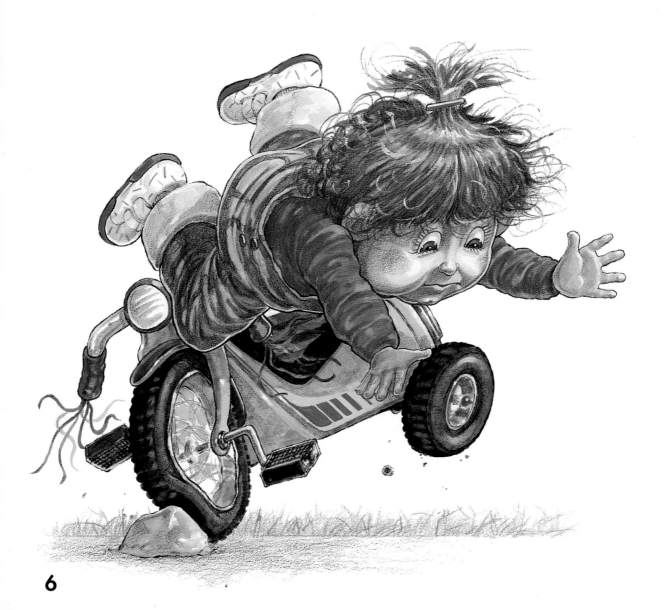

A bruise happens when small blood
vessels break. The blood stays
just under the top layer of my skin
and makes my skin look black and blue.

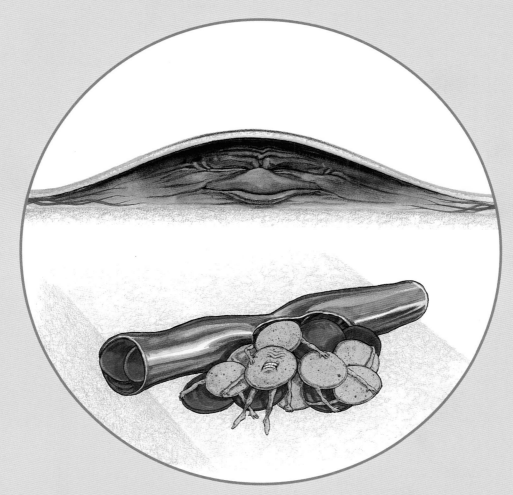

When I get a cut, blood comes out.
Soon the blood forms a clot
and the bleeding stops.
Then my skin makes new cells
to fill in the cut.

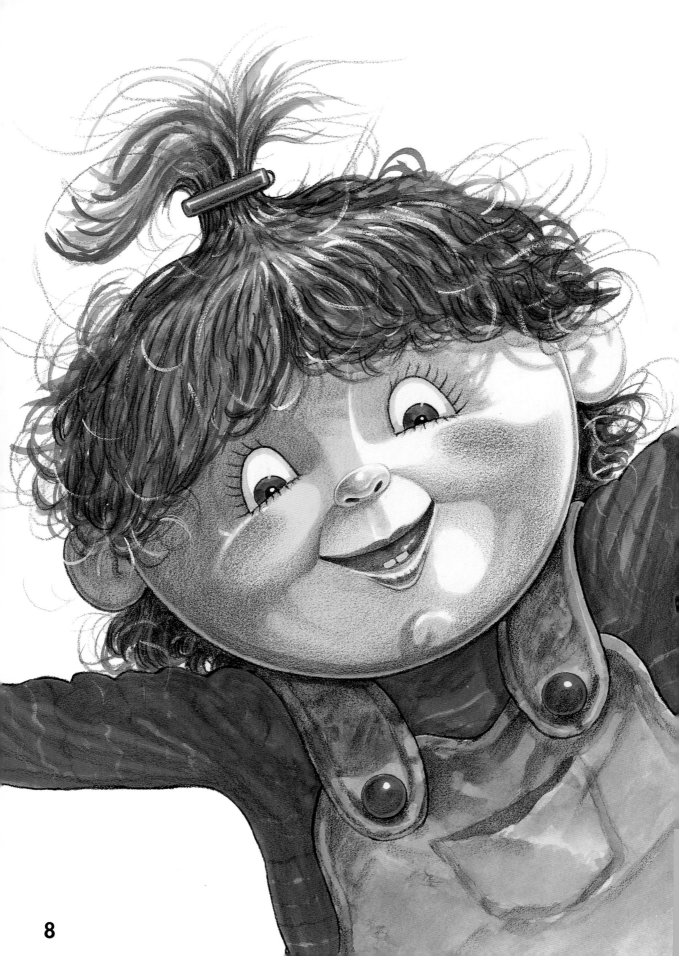

This is the **me**
that you can see.
But there's
so much more
inside of me!

My muscles help me climb a tree,
raise my arms, and lift my knee.
My muscles help me push and pull
and carry boxes that are full.

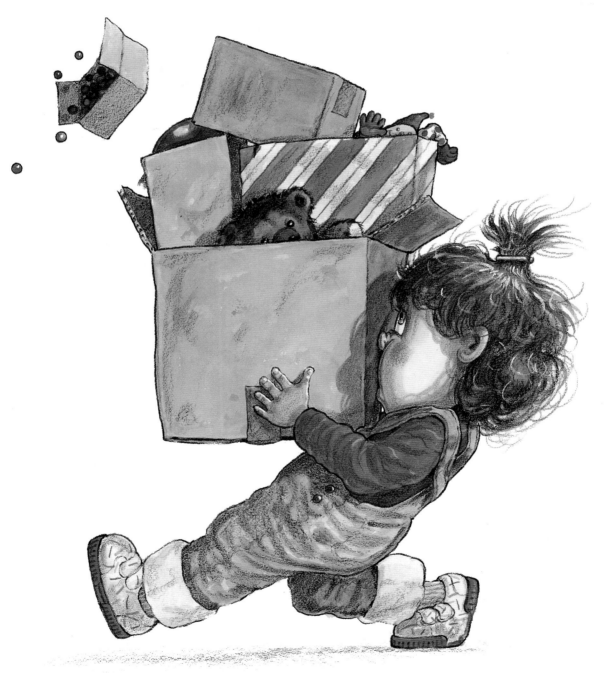

Muscles attached to my bones
help me move.
They stretch like rubber bands.
I can tell them when
I want them to work.
I use over 200 different muscles
just to walk.

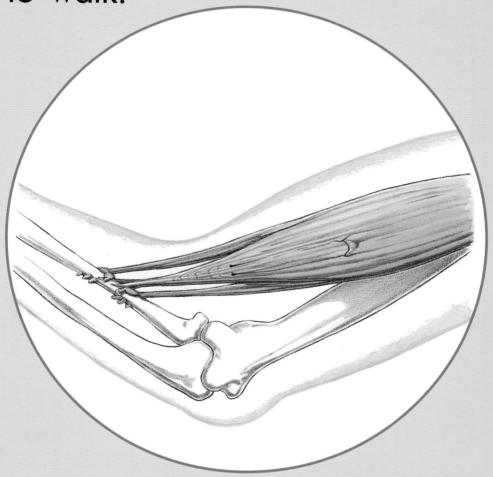

Sometimes my muscles get tired.
If I work and play too much,
I need to take a rest.

My muscles help me move about
and help my breath go in and out.

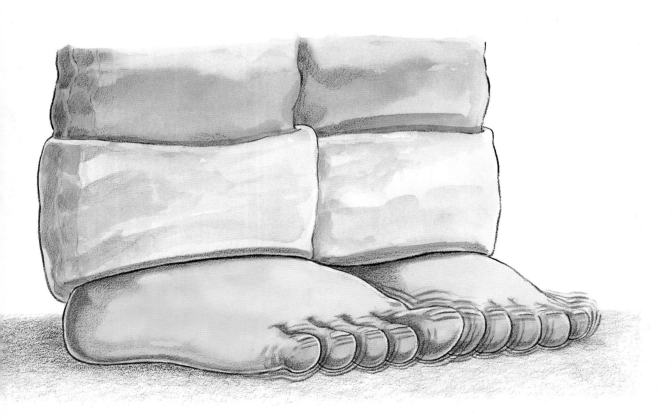

Muscles help me bend my toes,
and muscles help me blow my nose.

Some muscles inside of me
work by themselves.
These muscles work day and night
without me even telling them to.
Muscles help my lungs move air
in and out of my body so I can breathe.

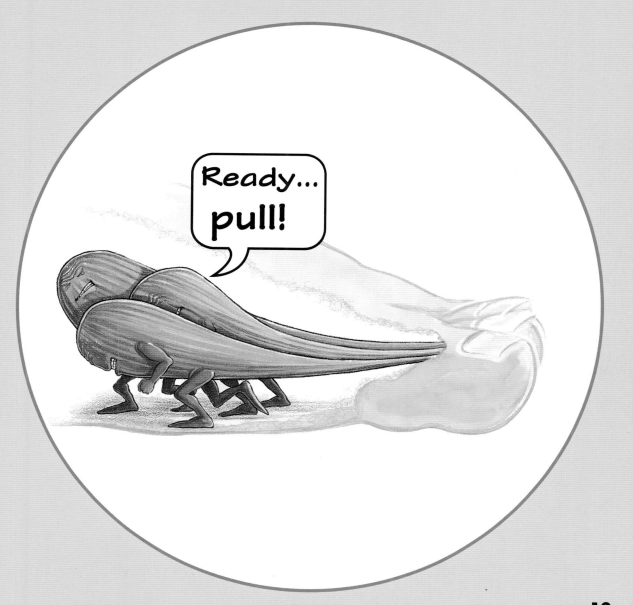

Muscles help me smile and wink
and swallow when I take a drink.
My muscles help me lift and throw,
and I can help my muscles grow!

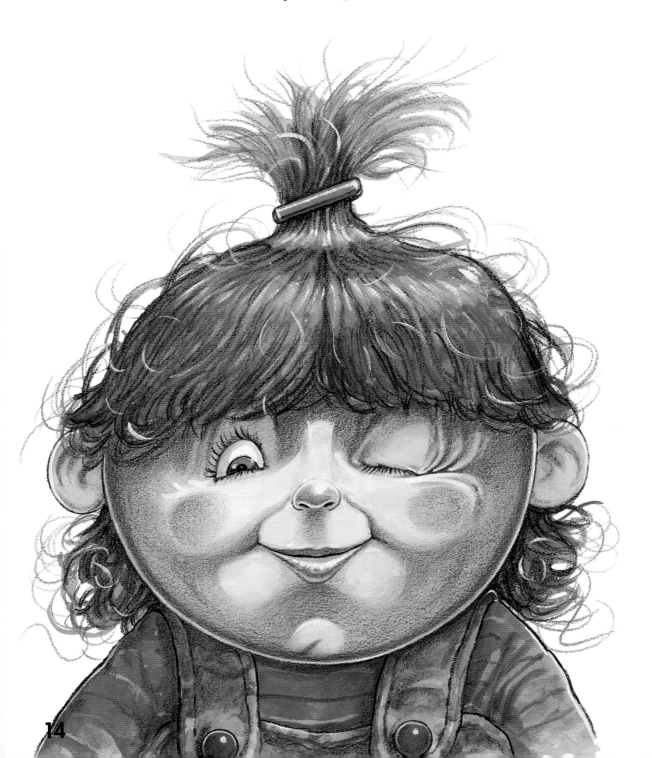

It takes 40 muscles to make a frown, but only 17 to make a smile. Without muscles, food and water could not move through my body.

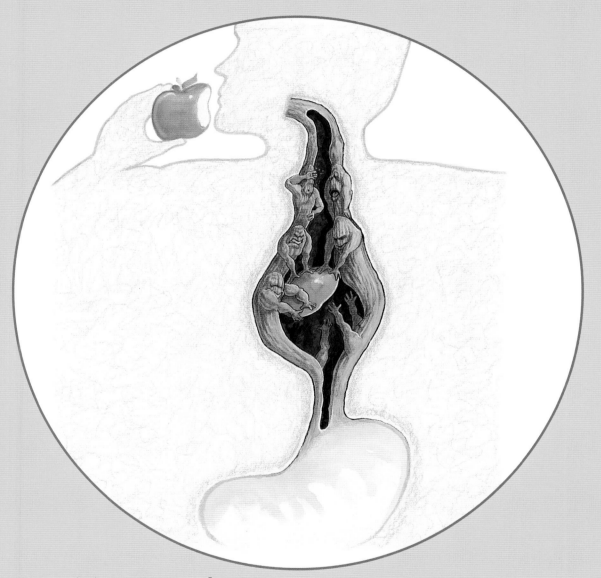

My muscles grow because I exercise, eat healthy foods, and get plenty of sleep.

This is the **me**
that you
can see.

But there's
so much more

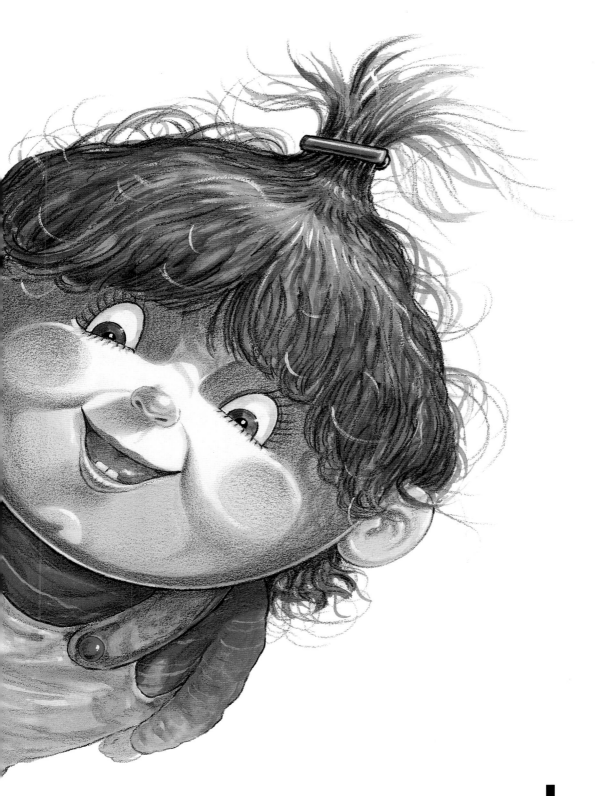

inside of me!

Bones are important, that's a fact.
They help my body stay intact.
I have 206 bones—to be exact!

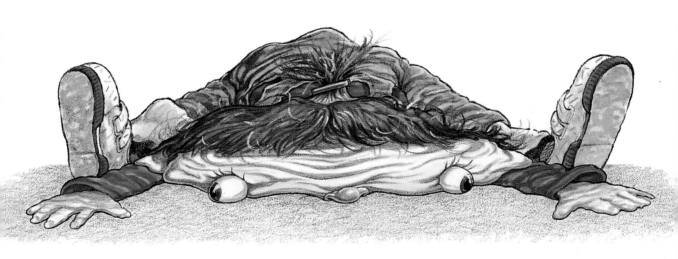

The bones I have I plan to keep.
Without them I'd be in a heap.

My bones are of many
shapes and sizes.
Some are long,
like in my arms and legs.
Some are round, like my ribs.
Some are short,
like in my hands and feet.

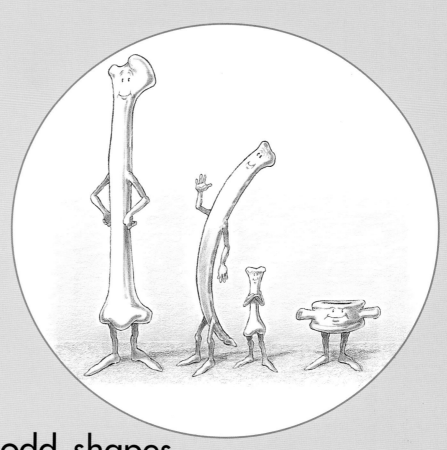

Some have odd shapes,
like my backbone.
Bones protect my lungs,
heart, and stomach.

I stand, I bend, I run, I jump.
Sometimes I fall and get a bump.
I'll bend my knees and elbows, too,
to show you what my joints can do!

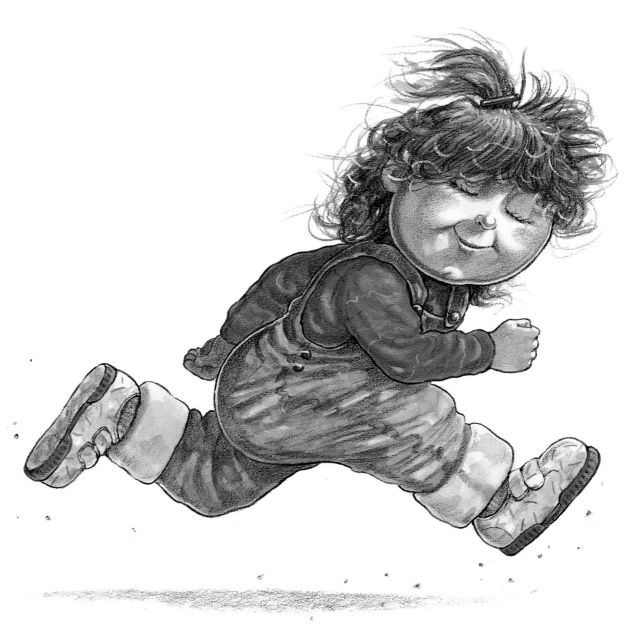

My joints are where my bones
meet each other.
I have many kinds of joints.
Some move a lot, and some
don't move at all.

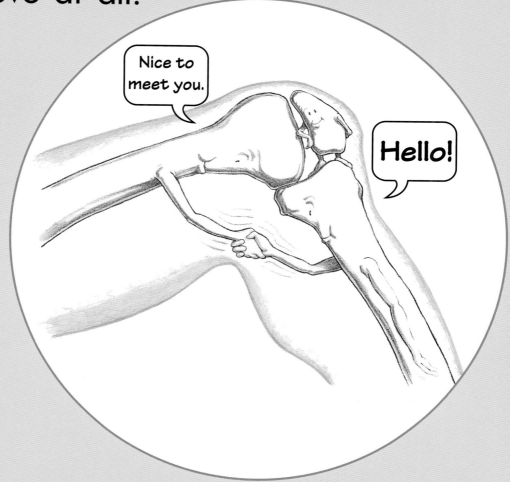

My bones, muscles, and joints
all work together
to let me twist and turn and jump.
It would be hard to jump
without bending my knee.

Bones help me to live and grow, and
even though it may seem slow,
I'm getting **bigger**...

Does it show????

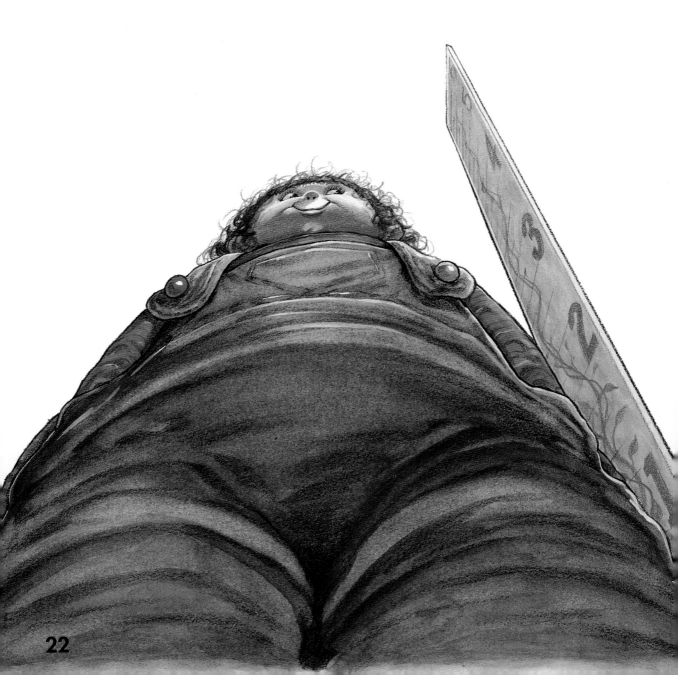

When my bones grow longer,
I grow taller.
All my bones together
form my skeleton.
My skeleton grows up with me.

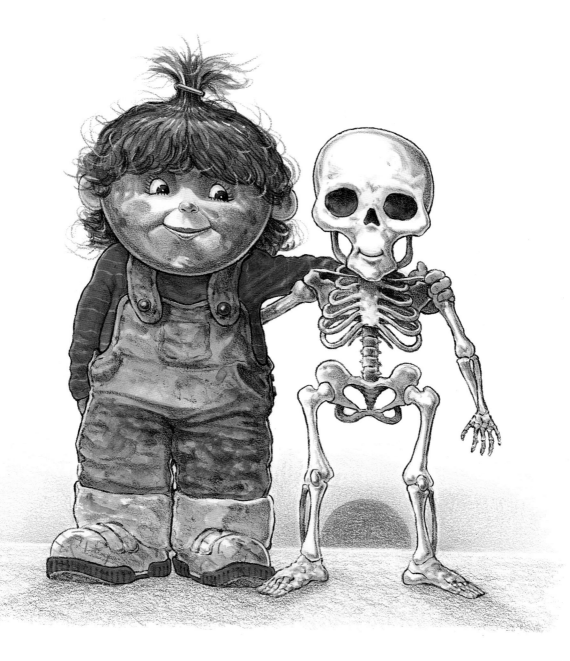

Muscles and bones,
bones and skin,
I like this body
that I'm in!

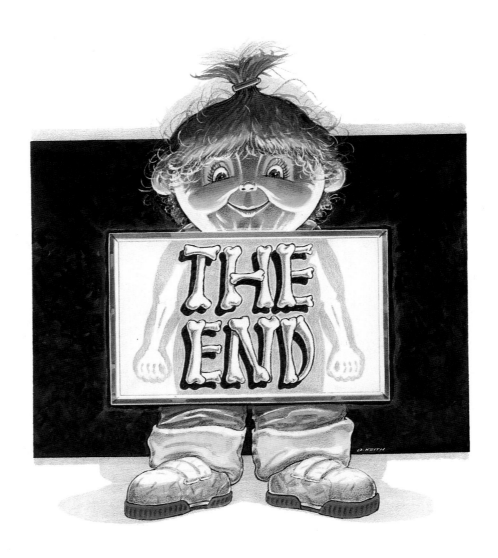